The Little
Book of
Yoga

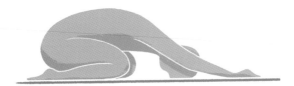

"Yoga is not a work-out,
it is a work-in."

Rolf Gates

The Little
Book of
Yoga

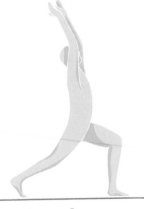

Lucy Lucas

An Hachette UK Company
www.hachette.co.uk

First published in Great Britain in 2019 by Gaia Books,
an imprint of Octopus Publishing Group Ltd

Carmelite House
50 Victoria Embankment
London EC4Y 0DZ
www.octopusbooks.co.uk

Distributed in the US by Hachette Book Group,
1290 Avenue of the Americas, 4th and 5th Floors, New York, NY 10104

Distributed in Canada by Canadian Manda Group
664 Annette Street, Toronto, Ontario, Canada M6S 2C8

ISBN 978-1-85675-399-9
A CIP catalogue record for this book is available from the British Library.

Printed and bound in China.
10 8 6 4 2 1 3 5 7 9

Publishing Director Stephanie Jackson
Art Director Juliette Norsworthy
Senior Editor Alex Stetter
Design and illustrations Abi Read
Senior Production Controller Allison Gonsalves

Contents

Introduction

What is Yoga?

Today about 300 million people around the world practise yoga. But what is it that we are practising? Yoga in the 21st century is predominantly a physical practice: a series of poses and postures, or *asanas* in Sanskrit, with a focus on the breath and an element of mindfulness – paying attention while moving. However, yoga was first mentioned in Sanskrit scriptures dating back to *c.*500 BCE.

While the idea of yoga as a practice makes sense to us today, the ancient Sanskrit texts focused on the outcome of these practices: deep relaxation, a quiet mind, a change of consciousness and a relationship with the surrounding world. Furthermore, in Sanskrit – the ancient language of India – the word *yoga* has many meanings. It can mean joining or attaching, as well as a method, trick, business, wealth, mixing, ordering, suitability, diligence or magic. Normally you will hear yoga teachers talk about the first of these meanings – to "join together" – but the variety of uses reflects the variety found within the practice of yoga.

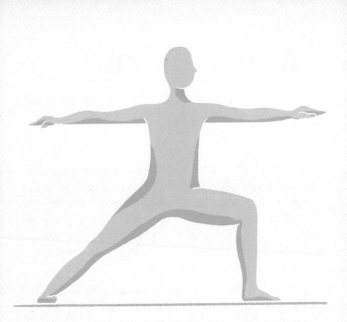

Nowadays people often take up yoga to improve flexibility and reduce stress, so these might be considered our desired outcomes, but they are far removed from the yogic states of *moksha* (liberation) and *samadhi* (meditative consciousness) described in various yogic texts. Yet, even its modern form, yoga gives us tools to examine our relationship with our bodies, ourselves and the world around us, and from there an opportunity to explore and understand the human condition. Anyone who has lain in Savasana (see page 78) at the end of a yoga class will have had a glimpse of the meditative yogic state described in those texts, and people often talk about their class enabling them to face the rest of the week in a different frame of mind. This is all yoga.

As our yoga practice develops, and we take more time just to be in the body and with the breath, we start to explore further this idea of being human, and how we live in this world. Many practitioners and teachers have stories of life changes that were catalyzed by yoga, and many more talk of how yoga helps the week flow better. It is in the way we allow the practice and experience of yoga to influence our lives off the mat, and outside the studio, that we can start to see the outcomes that were originally spoken about.

History

Yoga is an aggregating tradition, meaning that as new practices developed some of the older ideas were still being used. This is why some ideas about meditation, fasting, energy body practices and exploring altered states of consciousness from the Sramana movement of ancient India (dating back to around 600–300 BCE), plus those from Samkhya, another Indian philosophy, are found in the early Upanishad texts (700–100 BCE) and later in the famous *Bhagavadgita* in 300 CE.

Patanjali's *Yoga Sutras*, compiled before 400 CE, contain one or two sentences about how to sit and about the breath, but the text is primarily about the process and state of meditation. While Samkhyan philosophy was about transcending our impure, flawed existence, around 500 CE we see the rise of Tantric yoga, which emphasized how our true nature is simply perfect – we just don't know it.

From about 1300 CE onward, simplified ascetic and renunciate practices formed the basis of Hatha yoga. This added more postures, breathing exercises and bodily practices aimed at purity, and retained certain ideas from Tantra. Dating from the 1400s, the main Hatha yoga text, the *Hatha Yoga Pradipika*, was the first to include postures, or *asanas*, that we would recognize today. Adepts of Hatha yoga were mainly wandering men, who were feared because of some of their strange practices.

When the British arrived in India, it was these wandering Hatha *yogis* that they encountered, among numerous other religious and spiritual adherents. The *yogis* were viewed with distrust by the British and by many locals, although many of their practices continued throughout the colonial period into the 20th century.

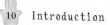

Yoga in the 20th & 21st Centuries

The father of modern postural yoga was Tirumalai Krishnamacharya (1888–1989), who was asked by the King of Mysore to develop a practice to strengthen the body and mind. Set against a context of anti-colonialism and Indian nationalism, the aim was to create a strong, independent Indian man.

Krishnamacharya borrowed heavily: from Swedish gymnastic calisthenics, other Western movement practices and Hatha yoga. Four of his students – K Pattabhi Jois, BKS Iyengar, TKV Desikachar and Indra Devi – went on to develop their own schools of yoga.

Western interest in yogic practices started to grow during the counter-cultural movement of the 1960s, with The Beatles famously visiting an *ashram*, or religious retreat, in northern India in 1968. As 21st-century life has become more hectic, stressful and overwhelming, so yoga has entered the mainstream. Used more as a therapeutic tool than a spiritual path, postural yoga and meditation are now easily accessible across Europe and North America.

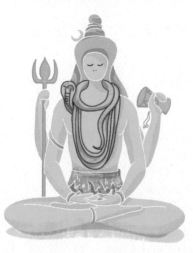

Yoga and Hinduism

Hinduism has come to mean the collective of all the traditions and sects that regard the Veda texts as the ultimate source of spiritual authority. But modern Hinduism is as much a cultural identity as a religious one. Today's yoga practitioner does not need to adopt a Hindu cultural or religious identity. Some practices may be reserved for those from a particular caste or clan, but the practices outlined in this book and in most mainstream yoga schools can be used by anyone, of any religious background – or none.

The Philosophy of Yoga

If yoga mainly means the goal of practice, then what is that goal? In order to understand more about the outcomes in yoga, it helps to see how *yogis* conceptualize the world.

Some schools of Indian philosophy are Dualist, in that they see the Supreme Self as being separate from the individual: the idea of God on a cloud. Non-Dualists see both the Supreme and the individual existing together as one reality: everything in this world is divine including us, we are simply one aspect of Reality becoming aware of itself. For example, Patanjali and the Samkhyans viewed the material world as dirty and flawed, and as something to be transcended to reach the Supreme. In contrast, many Tantrics saw the world as a manifestation of the divine, and the body as something to be embraced.

Both approaches require an awakening of awareness in the individual. Over the course of yoga's history, different groups have been creating and adapting a variety of practices designed to raise awareness of who we really are. This includes allowing life force (*prana*) to flow through us, removing our illusions (*malas*), unwinding our conditioning (*samskara*), quieting fluctuations of the mind (*vrttis*), improving concentration (*dharana*), unblocking energy centres (*chakras*) and awakening our true potential (*shakti*).

Practices included meditation, mantras (chanting), energy work with the breath (*pranayama*) and visualization, cleansing practices, and ethical and moral guidance for living (*yamas*, *niyamas*).

Postural yoga can be seen in a similar fashion: designed to release stuck energy in a physical way and grow an innate awareness of our physical selves.

1.

Postural Yoga

The Benefits of Modern Postural Yoga

Modern Postural Yoga has a number of health benefits, such as greater joint stability and mobility, an increased range of movement, improved bone and muscle strength, greater lung capacity and, depending on the style of yoga that is practised, cardiovascular benefits.

Yoga also improves our experience of stress by calming the nervous system and allowing us to spend more time in our "rest and restore" mode. This effect on the nervous system is said to have a wide range of benefits, from lower blood pressure to improved immunity.

Meditative, mindful and breathing practices can also help with calming the nervous system, and with a number of specific techniques designed to reduce emotional reactivity, improve mood and process difficult feelings and reactions.

As a spiritual tradition, yoga can bring a greater sense of self-awareness and connectedness to ourselves, others and the world around us. For some people, this may simply bring about a greater sense of wellbeing, while for others it may create a profound shift in how they experience reality.

Common Misconceptions

You do not have to be bendy or thin to practise yoga. You do not have to be flexible, either, but if you aren't, you may want to use props to help you. Despite what you might see on social media, yoga isn't particularly difficult: most people are not practising advanced poses. The wide and ever-growing number of yoga styles means that everyone can find something that suits their needs and temperament.

Don't let the spiritual and philosophical tradition of yoga put you off. In a physical class, many teachers will not mention them at all, or only briefly: take from the class whatever means the most to you.

The Right Kind of Yoga for You

There are so many different kinds of yoga that finding a type that suits you can feel overwhelming. This section provides an overview of the main kinds of yoga you will come across.

Ashtanga

Ashtanga yoga is a set series of poses devised by K Pattabhi Jois (see page 11). The poses are linked together with a shortened Sun Salutation sequence called a *vinyasa*.

In a teacher-led Ashtanga class, students follow the sequence of poses together. In a Mysore-style class, students follow the series by themselves and the teacher helps where necessary, allowing students to progress at their own speed.

Ashtanga is a vigorous form of postural yoga, best suited to those with a good level of fitness. The benefits can be those of a moving meditation, where the mind is quiet as the body moves through the poses. Cardiovascular fitness can also be improved. However, the constant repetition may cause issues in the body, particularly in the knees and shoulders.

Vinyasa

Derived from the Ashtanga system of moving from pose to pose with the breath, Vinyasa yoga doesn't follow a standard sequence, thereby allowing teachers greater creativity in their classes. It includes types such as flow, dynamic, power, rocket, Baptiste and Jivamukti yoga.

Sequences are arranged around Sun Salutations (see page 92), with variations added to the core poses; or may include a series of postures interspersed with shortened Sun Salutations.

Vinyasa classes are great for a sense of freedom and flow, raising the heart rate and promoting the role of the breath. The movement will create heat in the body, which can alleviate stiffness and immobility, although this needs to be managed with awareness.

In faster classes the teacher will have little time to instruct how to do a pose or check that students are following it correctly. Dynamic classes require a degree of physical fitness and flexibility. A slow-flow class, with time to get into postures, make adjustments and find the breath, is better for a beginner.

Hatha

All physical yoga practices are Hatha yoga, as this refers to the role the *asanas*, or poses, played in Hatha yoga from around 1400 to 1900 CE. Today, teachers and studios tend to use this term for slower, less dynamic classes, including those with greater focus on seated *pranayama* and meditation exercises.

These classes can be just as challenging as the more dynamic ones, because holding poses with stability and muscle engagement is not easy. The slower pace, however, can make them more appropriate for beginners, as there is time to come into the pose, find the alignment that fits your body and for the teacher to review what you are doing.

Similar classes might be called classical or traditional yoga; or they might be given a specific name, such as Sivananda.

Iyengar

BKS Iyengar was a student of Krishnamacharya in Mysore, along with K Pattabhi Jois of Ashtanga yoga fame (see page 18). Iyengar is a form of Hatha yoga, with a focus on alignment, control and precision. Students start with simple poses and progress to more complex ones over time. Iyengar yoga makes extensive use of props and equipment to assist students in exploring the poses.

Iyengar is not a dynamic practice, and its stillness can be great for developing awareness of the breath and the body, as well as for learning the individual *asanas* in detail. However, its precise, and sometimes strict, alignment principles may not work for certain individuals.

For a more dynamic practice, you could try Anusara yoga, which is based on similar but less precise principles and is more of a Vinyasa flow-style of yoga (see page 19).

Hot yoga

This type of yoga is practised in a room heated to 30–37°C (86–99°F). Any style of yoga can be practised in the heat, from Vinyasa to Hatha, but the most famous form of hot yoga is perhaps Bikram yoga, a set sequence of poses popularized by Bikram Choudhury.

Research shows that there are no benefits over doing yoga in a normal temperature, but hot yoga is popular because the heat can make us feel more flexible and open in our bodies. While pleasant, this can encourage over-extending and over-stretching. This can be avoided by mindfully staying away from your end-range of movement, which can be greater in the heat. Your heart and lungs may also work harder, providing cardiovascular benefits, although there is a chance of stressing the body as if it is doing a high-intensity workout. None of this makes hot yoga a problem, but it does require good body awareness.

In a hot yoga class, you will sweat – a lot! If heat makes you feel flustered, stressed or overwhelmed, it might be best to avoid it.

Restorative & Yin yoga

People tend either to love restorative yoga – or its cousin,
Yin yoga – or hate it. These forms of yoga ask us to be still
and quiet, with no distractions except what is going on for
us in that moment: physically, mentally and emotionally.
Without movement to focus on, it can be difficult to just
"be". These practices are excellent for developing inner
awareness, as well as for relaxation and rest.

In restorative yoga,
poses are usually
floor-based and use lots
of props, to ensure the
body is fully supported.
Poses can be held for
five to ten minutes, and
the teacher will often
guide meditations or
gentle breathing
exercises, or read poems
during this time.

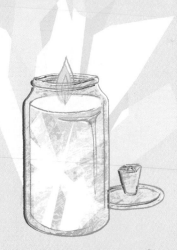

Yin yoga aims to allow the muscles to relax and then adds stress to other tissues: ligaments, tendons, fascia and joints. Poses are mainly floor-based and are held for two to five minutes, sometimes longer. It can be a restful practice, although sensation may be strong in a different way from a dynamic practice. Students are encouraged to keep on the softer side of their "edge" of sensation, and to resist the temptation to go deeper into a pose and risk injury. Yin is a great practice for working with awareness, and for noticing the desire in all of us to strive and reach. For this reason, it may not be suitable for complete beginners.

Yin yoga should be avoided in pregnancy, due to the impact on ligaments. Students with hypermobility should consult the teacher before attending a class.

2.
Practice

The Teacher

The teacher–student relationship has traditionally been central to yoga. Students would work one-on-one with their teacher or guru, and practices and knowledge would be passed down, until the student was considered experienced enough to be initiated into a particular lineage. It would take years to become a master.

Today anyone can sign up for a 200-hour teacher-training programme, which is considered the entry-level standard for a yoga instructor. But not all of these people will be good at teaching yoga. You might need to try several classes before you find the right teacher, but it will help your practice if you can find one from whom you really want to learn.

In a physical class, teachers may perform adjustments to help a student into a deeper version of the pose or correct their alignment. If you do not want to be touched or adjusted, let the teacher know at the start of the class.

A good yoga teacher will:

🤚 Provide some background concerning why you are there and what is happening in the class – some philosophy or theory, and some anatomical or therapeutic health advice.

🤚 Bring students into awareness of their bodies and their breath, as this embodiment is central to yoga.

🤚 Provide modifications for students with injuries or other health conditions (including not letting you take part in the class at all, if it's not suitable for you).

🤚 Encourage students to be mindful of their own limits and to back away from pain.

🤚 Set appropriate boundaries around timekeeping, mat space, availability for questions, physical touch and external relationships.

🤚 Include some aspects of meditation or *pranayama* (breath control, see page 36).

🤚 *Always* leave time for Savasana (see page 78).

Where to Practise

There are numerous places to practise yoga, and many people base their decision on logistics, but it's worth considering what you get in each setting.

Gyms & fitness clubs

Gyms and leisure centres are one of the first places many people will try yoga, often because classes are included in their membership. These classes tend to focus more on the *asanas*, or poses, than on meditation or *pranayama*, although this depends very much on the teacher. Some gym-based teachers will also be fitness instructors, which adds good knowledge to body work and movement, but may make the classes more vigorous.

Gym classes can be quite large, so it can be easy to get lost in the crowd. The slower and smaller the class, the better for beginners and those with injuries, as you will have time to come into the postures – and the teacher can watch you and make suggestions. Hiding at the back of a packed class may feel safe, but you could easily miss out on helpful instruction.

Yoga studios

Yoga studios come in all shapes and sizes, from multi-site behemoths to small local places with just a couple of teachers. They will typically be more expensive than a gym, especially if you pay per class as a drop-in student. But most will offer bulk-purchase discounts or even membership.

A good studio will usually have all the equipment you need, will be appropriately heated, will accurately describe classes and their suitability, and will take care over who they hire as teachers. Classes are often smaller than those at gyms, but this does depend on the studio.

If you are new to yoga, returning after a long absence or have an injury, look for classes aimed at beginners or labelled Level 1. A Level 2–3 class will include more advanced poses and will suit those with considerable experience and a good base fitness level. You may find that you can move on to different levels and styles of yoga as you become accustomed to the practice.

Other venues

Many yoga teachers supplement gym and studio classes with those they run independently in local halls, at festivals and even in workplaces. These venues might lack the "yoga vibe", especially in an office, where you might be lying next to a flipchart; and you may need to bring your own mat. The great thing about such classes is that yoga is brought close to you in your workplace or local community.

Private classes

An option for those who would like close attention from a teacher, to understand their body and yoga practice, is a private one-to-one session in your home or in a studio, or sometimes in the home of the teacher. Ensure that you feel comfortable being in a private space with the teacher, especially at home.

Private sessions are expensive, but a one-to-one relationship enables the teacher to really get to know you and your body, and to work toward meeting your needs. This can be good for those starting yoga or returning to it after injury, and who want to make sure of any modifications before joining a group class.

Online videos & apps

If you can't make it to a class, are on a tight budget or want to supplement classes, there are plenty of options online. These range from free videos on YouTube to a range of paid online systems. Online materials give so many options, from movement to meditation, from five minutes to two hours, so there is always something for your practice, if you require it.

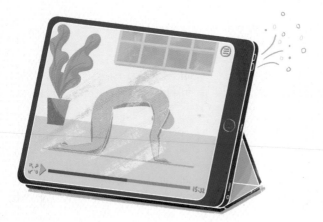

What to Wear

Contrary to popular belief, you don't need special clothing for yoga. You need to be comfortable in various positions: lying down, sitting and lunging. You need room to move, but nothing so baggy that it might get in the way, like a top that falls in your face when you're halfway upside down. If you are doing a rigorous practice, you don't want to overheat, but always bring an extra layer for Savasana, as the body can cool quickly when you are still. Private parts of the body need be adequately supported and covered.

As best you can, try practising with bare feet, as socks prevent correct activation of the feet and the muscle chain through the leg, into the pelvis. Regular socks can make you slide, causing a different muscular engagement pattern; or you might come to rely on the grippy soles of rubber-bottomed socks, rather than using your muscles.

Mats

You don't necessarily need a yoga mat. The floor will often do, especially if you're practising at home – with some blankets to support your knees, and for cosiness in Savasana. Most gyms and studios will provide mats for students to use.

If you buy a mat, note that it should provide some cushioning, but should not be so soft that you cannot feel the floor underneath. If a mat is too squishy, it is harder for you to push away the floor and create a feedback loop of muscular energy. If your knees are unhappy when you are on all fours, fold the mat over to double the thickness, or use a blanket or cushion.

Using Props

Props such as blocks, bricks, cushions, bolsters, straps and blankets are your friends. You can use them to cushion and support your body, to find extra space in a pose or to make a pose more comfortable and available to you. Yoga studios will usually have a range of equipment for you to use, and the teacher should encourage use of them when required. Gyms and other venues may not necessarily have a full range of kit, and in large classes it may more difficult for a teacher to notice individuals who need extra support. Getting to know what works for *you* is key.

And remember: using props does not mean that you are "bad" at yoga.

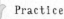

3.

Breath

Breathing Correctly

The breath is central to the practice of yoga, both physical and meditative yoga. *Yogis* use the power of the breath – as the only major life process in our body that is both conscious and unconscious – to tap into the unconscious. We can also manipulate the breath to help us improve our wellbeing.

Many people do not breathe fully or correctly. Several things can affect the quality of our breathing: muscle strength and flexibility, lung capacity, what's going on emotionally, as well as illness and injury. If we are not breathing fully, we cannot be fully oxygenated, leading to fatigue, anxiety and lethargy.

Physical yoga helps, as we have to breathe in order to move. Breathing while in the postures strengthens and lengthens our breathing capacity, while breathing when still makes us more aware of *how* we breathe. As our breath is linked to the nervous system, we can help to calm ourselves by calming the breath; this can also help to still the mind. Breathing techniques are often used as a gateway to meditation.

All physical yoga should include at least a few minutes of "breath attention", when you focus solely on the mechanics of your breathing. Some classes might include specific breathing techniques. Remember that everyone breathes differently, so if your breathing is slightly different from your teacher's, don't worry. Just keep breathing in your own way – and don't hold your breath.

The three breathing techniques on the following pages can be done alone or sequentially, for a longer practice.

Take your time!

Breath Attention

1 Lie down with the knees bent, and perhaps with a cushion under the knees.

2 Bring one hand onto your navel and one onto your chest.

3 Allow your breath to settle into its natural pattern and rhythm. Breathe through your nose.

4 Start to notice the following, with a curious, nonjudgmental mind:

🤚 Is the breath long, short or somewhere in the middle? Is the inhale different from the exhale?

🤚 Is the breath deep or shallow, or in between?

🤚 Is the breath jagged or smooth, or are the in-breath and out-breath different?

🤚 Is each breath coming fast or slow? What is the frequency of the breath?

🤚 Can you feel where the inhale starts in your body? Where does it stop? How about the exhale?

🤚 Where do you most feel your breath? In the belly? The chest? The nostrils?

Banana Breathing

1 Lie down with the legs extended and the ankles wide, then take your arms overhead.

2 Hold onto the right wrist with the left hand and take your arms, shoulders and torso over toward the left.

3 Cross your right ankle over your left, so that you make a banana shape on the floor.

4 Notice what happens to your breathing. Can you send your breath more into the right-hand side of your torso, inflating the right lung and moving the muscles between the right-side ribs?

5 Repeat on the other side, noting any differences.

Full Yogic Breath

A full yogic breath means fully activating the diaphragm, the muscle that enables breathing, and filling all of your lung capacity.

1 Lie flat again, with one hand on the navel and one on the chest.

2 As you breathe in, allow the tummy to expand away from the spine, creating room for the diaphragm to move down and the lungs to open.

3 Continue your inhale into the side of the ribcage, up under the armpits. If it is comfortable, allow the inhale to continue into the upper chest, maybe slightly elevating the collar bones.

4 To exhale, follow the directions in reverse order: the upper chest exhales, the ribs empty and the belly sinks down to the spine, allowing the diaphragm to move up and "push" any remaining air out of the lungs.

5 The inhale and exhale should not be forced. It may take several rounds of breath, or even several practices, before you feel comfortable opening the upper chest. Take your time and allow the breath to do its own work.

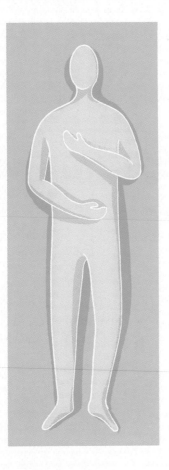

Pranayama

Often misinterpreted as just breathing, *pranayama* is integral
to how *yogis* manage energy in the body.

Prana is universal energy, or life force, which is everywhere.
When it flows into us, it makes us feel alive and energetic.
Pranayama is the balancing of this energy inside and outside
the body. If we have too much *prana* outside, we can feel
restless, flaky or worried. If we don't have enough *prana*
inside, we can feel aimless, stuck or fatigued.

Our bodies are often full of unwanted "stuff", such as
physical tension or emotional and psychological belief
patterns that are holding us back, which means there isn't
room for *prana* to enter. Many *yogis*, going back thousands
of years, have used *pranayama* to free up such blockages.
It can also be used to cool and calm the nervous system, as
well as to direct energies around the body. You may have had
the experience of something "shifting" after a yoga class.

Beginners should approach *pranayama* with caution.
Some techniques – such as Kapabalati, Bashtrika and breath
retention – are advanced practices that can have strong
effects. If you are interested in *pranayama*, then a course or
workshop with a teacher with specialist training in this field
is a good starting point.

Five types of prana

- Prana Vayu: works to bring *prana* into the body, on the inhale.

- Apana Vayu: works to release "stuff" from the body, on the exhale.

- Samana Vayu: works with the belly and solar plexus to generate fire and energy.

- Vyana Vayu: works to circulate *prana* throughout the body.

- Udana Vayu: works to move *prana* upward.

Simple *pranayama*:
ujjayi or ocean breath

This is a calming breathing technique you can do in a seated posture or while moving in a physical practice.

1 Bring the tip of your tongue to the roof of the mouth, just behind the teeth.

2 Close the lips and start to breathe through your nose. The slight closing of the throat allows the breath to make an "ocean" sound as it travels through the nose and throat.

The effect is to calm and soothe the breath, which in turn calms the nervous system. The ocean sound should be soft – be careful not to turn into Darth Vader, especially in a physical practice.

Another simple *pranayama* technique is Nadi Shodhana (see page 88).

4.

Meditation & Mindfulness

Types of Meditation

Meditation is one of the earliest yoga practices. The word can be used to describe both a state of consciousness (*samadhi*) and the techniques that work toward it. This state can involve experiencing a change in consciousness, greater awareness, presence, connection to the universe and our true nature.

Meditation may be taught as part of a regular yoga class or separately. There are many different kinds, from differing traditions, so it can be helpful to understand the various types of meditation and what they might be used for. Many types are Buddhist in origin, while others come from Indian spiritual traditions such as Vedanta and Saiva Tantra. More modern forms of meditation, such as mindfulness, are based on older practices, often with the spiritual element removed.

Concentration

This involves focusing on one object while allowing everything else to fade into the background. The object of meditation may be outside the body, such as a candle flame, or inside, such as the breath or a mantra (chanted sounds or words). A more subtle version would be to focus on energy centres, or *chakras*, in the body.

Awareness

Awareness includes mindful practices, such as mindful eating or walking; sitting with awareness of the breath; and awareness of being aware. Many of these practices have a self-inquiry element. Yoga Nidra – sometimes called "yogic sleep" – works in a similar fashion, by guiding your awareness to particular parts of the body.

Integrative meditation

This involves holding your attention on an object, and then just being with whatever arises. Many modern mindfulness meditations are based on this technique.

Other kinds of meditation include contemplation, such as on a word or a piece of text, as well as self-talk processes and visualizations such as "going on a journey".

How to Meditate

Sit, close the eyes and watch your breath.

This is one of the simplest, and yet most difficult, meditation practices! If you attempt this, you'll notice that your mind intrudes or wanders off, even after just one or two breaths. So it's helpful to have a guide or to know some techniques, which essentially give the "monkey mind" a job to do. There are some short concentration-based meditations in this book (see pages 82 and 90), which take only five to ten minutes to complete.

If you are unsure how to proceed, here are some other ideas:

 Use an app or a video to guide you: there are many options available for modern mindfulness-based practices, such as apps that have guided meditations as well as timers with gongs and bells to keep you present.

 Take a course, either online or in person.

 Join a local meditation group: your local Buddhist centre would be a good place to start, or perhaps a local studio. Check the instructor's credentials with your yoga teacher. Meditation is not widely taught on introductory yoga teacher-training, and ideally meditation teachers should have had further training.

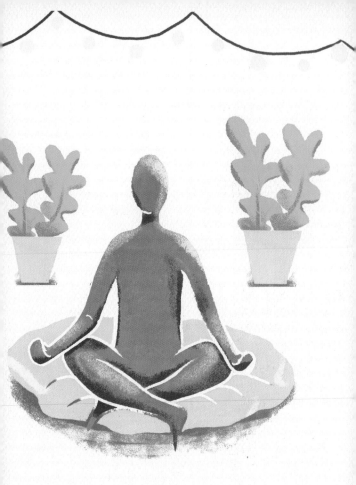

Meditation & Physical Yoga

You can bring meditative elements into your physical yoga practice in a couple of ways.

Mindful movement: As you practise, bring your awareness to your body, focusing less on the shapes you make or how you look and more on how it *feels*. When you are being still in a pose, focus on your breath.

Use movement to still the body and mind: Movement releases physical, mental and emotional tension, so that sitting in stillness becomes easier on the body and the mind. In Savasana (see page 78), see if you can stay present with the breath and/or the sensations in the body, and allow any thoughts to move to the background of your awareness.

Meditation and mental health

Meditation is held up as a panacea for many things, but it is not always calming, or even helpful. Many people feel irritated, bored or anxious when meditating. More importantly, if you have a mental-health diagnosis, then as well as speaking to your doctor, you need to inform your meditation teacher so that they can advise you.

5. Poses

1

TADASANA
Mountain Pose

This is a wonderful way to find stillness and stability in the body. Mountain Pose is like a standing meditation: see if you can stand, relax and breathe.

1 Stand upright with your arms by your side and your weight distributed equally through both legs. Some styles of yoga expect the feet to be together in this pose, but you may feel more stable with the feet further apart, so adjust the distance to find a comfortable position. Put more weight into the outside edge of the feet and heels, keeping the balls and toes in contact with the floor.

2 Soften the knees, so that the knee joint is not locked. If you notice your knees rolling in toward each other, put more weight into the outside edge of the foot. Close your eyes and shift your weight from foot to foot, until you feel your pelvis is completely supported by your legs.

3 Focus on your torso. Are you puffing out your chest, rounding your shoulders or sticking out your buttocks? Gently move the spine until you feel equal space in front of and behind the body. Allow your weight to drop into your feet, and find your breath.

Benefits

 Improves balance.

 Increases awareness of the relationship between the feet, legs and hips.

Modifications

 If balance is an issue, stand near a wall or chair for support or do a seated variation.

 This pose may cause dizziness if held for a long time, especially if you have low blood pressure.

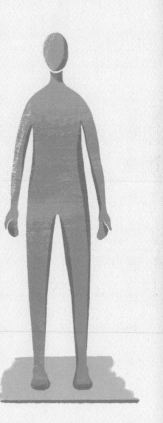

UTTANASANA
Forward Fold

This is a gentle, calming release for the back, as you let gravity work on lengthening the spine.

1 From standing, bend the knees and start to roll down the spine. Tuck in your chin, roll your shoulders forward and round through the back, until you get a slight hinge at the hips.

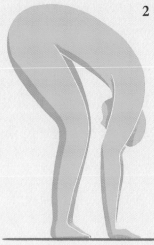

2 Place your hands on the floor, if possible, or a block or chair. Shift your weight from foot to foot, and adjust the distance between them so it feels comfortable. Put more weight into the outside edge of the feet and heels, keeping the balls and toes in contact with the floor.

3 Keep the knees bent and the tummy toward the thighs. The head should feel heavy and your gaze should be roughly between your knees.

4 As you breathe in, lengthen the front of your body slightly; with each exhale, soften a little more into the pose.

5 To come out of the pose, roll up, keeping the chin tucked in and the hips over the ankles until you're standing.

Benefits

 Releases the hamstrings, as well as opening the calves and hips. The bent knees release the lower back.

Modifications

 With lower back pain, headaches or low blood pressure: keep the back flat and the chest lifted, placing the hands on a block, wall or chair. Do not roll up or down: keep the navel pulled toward the spine, as you hinge from the hips to come up or down. Keep the knees bent.

 For tight hamstrings: keep the knees bent.

MARJARIASANA & BITILASANA

3 Cat & Cow

This combination of coordinated movement, breathing and awareness is an excellent warm-up, as well as a great way to reset the spine after one-sided sequences or lunges.

1 On all fours, shift the weight between your hands and knees; adjust until you feel your body is fully supported. Soften the elbows; take weight into the outside and heel of the hands, with fingers and thumbs connecting to the floor.

2 Connect to the sensation dragging your hands slightly away from you, to lift the chest and tailbone and look forward. This is Cow Pose.

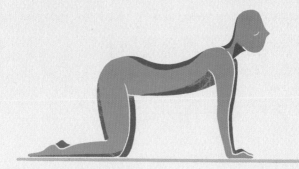

3 Push the hands down and pull them slightly inward, as if pushing the floor away. This allows you to round your back and shoulders, bring your gaze to your belly button and drop your tailbone. This is Cat Pose. Avoid bending the elbow as you move, but keep the elbow joints soft.

4 Move between the two poses in time to your own breath. Pay attention to the almost wave-like quality of the spine as it moves between flexion (Cow) and extension (Cat).

Benefits

 Actively stretches the back, torso and neck, improving spinal alignment. Can also help with back pain.

Modifications

 If you have pain in the wrists or shoulders, do the flexion and extension of the spine while seated.

 If the knees are painful, use padding.

BALASANA
Child's Pose

This resting pose lengthens the spine and opens the hips.

1 On all fours, move your hips back to your heels and bring your forehead toward the floor.

2 On each inhale, direct your breath into your back: to the kidney area, ribs and shoulder blades.

3 On each exhale, allow your head and tailbone to become heavy. Avoid pushing; simply relax on each exhale.

4 Knees can be close together or wide, with big toes touching.

Benefits

🖐 Restorative, calming and brings attention to the breath.

🖐 Useful as a rest pose at any point during a class, or as an alternative to Down Dog (see page 60).

Modifications

🖐 For painful knees: bring the hips forward to release the pressure, or place a rolled-up mat or cushion between the heels and the hips.

🖐 If coming forward to the floor is uncomfortable, keep the head lifted, resting it on your hands, a block or a large cushion.

5 ADHO MUKHA SVANASANA
Down Dog

One of the most famous poses in postural yoga, this mild inversion can be quite calming.

1 On all fours, walk your hands out in front of you until your arms are straight. Move the hips back, until the spine feels long.

2 Tuck your toes under and push through the heels to lift the knees off the ground. Adjust the distance between your hands and feet to support your body weight. Keep the weight on the outside edge and heel of the hands. Feel the connection up the arms into the side of your torso. Keep the head and neck soft, and your gaze on your belly.

3 Keep the knees soft and, with each exhale, lengthen the tailbone backward. Nothing should be locked or straining. You can move in Down Dog by pedalling the feet, moving the hips from side to side or lifting one leg.

Benefits

🖐 An upper-body strengthener that also opens the shoulders, calves, hamstrings and hands.

Modifications

🖐 If you have tight hamstrings, bend your knees.

🖐 If you have weak shoulders or wrists or lack strength, do Crouching Puppy: on your hands and knees, tuck the toes under and move your hips back toward your heels. Extend your arms away from you, so that they are active and the elbows are lifted off the floor. Engage the hands, side-body and tailbone as you would in Down Dog.

6

Low Lunge & High Lunge

These lunges open the hips and strengthen the glutes while
also working the torso and core.

Low Lunge

1 On all fours, step the right foot forward, just to the
outside of your right hand.

2 Shift the weight onto the outside edge and heel of the
front (right) foot, while keeping the toes connected to
the floor.

3 Push through the foot and lift the chest into a vertical
position. You can push your hands against your thigh to
help lift the chest, if necessary. Position the front foot so
that you can push firmly straight down through the heel
into the floor.

4 Bring the arms up alongside the ears, keeping the
shoulders and neck relaxed.

5 Lengthen through the sides of the torso, ensuring that
your shoulders don't come up by your ears.

6 Repeat with the left leg leading.

Benefits

 Both Low Lunge and High Lunge work the hips and thighs, bringing stability.

 Strengthens the glutes and encourages the hips to open.

Modifications

 If the back knee is uncomfortable on the floor, use a blanket for cushioning.

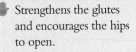

CONTINUES OVERLEAF...

For a stronger version, you can move from Low Lunge into High Lunge, as follows:

High Lunge

1 Starting in Low Lunge, bring your hands to the floor, tuck the back toes under and lift the back knee from the floor. Position your back foot so that you can push firmly through the heel and feel supported.

2 Push down through your front foot to lift the chest; you can push your hands against your thigh. Once the chest is lifted, you can reposition your back foot so that you feel more stable. Try bringing it closer to the front foot, or taking it wider, if you feel wobbly.

3 Keep the weight on the big toe, outside edge and heel of the front foot. The back foot should be balanced on the ball and toes, with the heel lifted. Keep the back knee bent or soft: there should be a sense of lightness in the pose.

4 Raise your arms up by your ears, with the neck and shoulders staying soft.

Benefits

 Activates the core, especially when the arms are raised.

Modifications

 If the sensation in the hips is too strong, shorten the distance between the back and front knees/legs.

 If you experience back pain in High Lunge, keep more of a bend in the back knee.

VIRABHADRASANA 2
7 Warrior 2

This is one of several yoga poses named after the fierce warrior Virabhadra, an incarnation of the god Siva.

1 From Mountain Pose (see page 52), step back with your right foot and press the heel down and the toes out, so that the foot is flat.

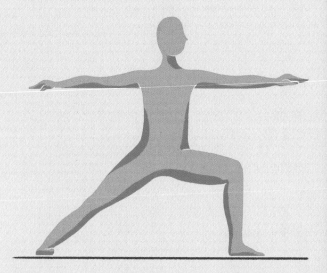

2 Keeping the front foot pointing forward, bend into the front knee. Keep the back leg straight. Adjust the distance between the feet, if necessary, until this feels comfortable. Avoid the front knee overshooting the ankle.

3 Bring your arms up parallel at shoulder height; activate the hands and fingers and reach them slightly away from you. Keep the neck and shoulders soft. Your chest should be open to the side, and your gaze over the front hand.

4 Connect the heels and toes to the floor, then transition the weight onto the outside edge of the feet. Explore drawing the inner thighs toward each other to engage the leg muscles.

Benefits

🖐 Opens the hips and strengthens the legs, glutes and arms.

🖐 Generates energy and fighting spirit.

Modifications

🖐 If new to the pose: temper the depth of the lunge over the front knee or take the feet wider.

🖐 For stiff necks: look in any direction that is comfortable.

🖐 For arm and shoulder issues: leave the hands on the hips.

8

VRKSASANA
Tree Pose

An important pose for working on balance and breath.

1 From standing, shift your weight onto the left leg
   and soften the knee.

2 Bring your right foot up against your calf or thigh,
   with the toes pointing down. Keep the hips facing
   forward and the standing knee soft.

3 Find a focal point to rest your gaze upon, to help
   your stability.

4 Engage your core by drawing the belly button
   toward the spine.

5 Bring your hands into the prayer position in front
   of the chest.

6 If you feel stable, you can bring the arms up
   alongside your ears.

Benefits

🖐 Great for practising balance and finding stillness.

Modifications

🖐 For tight hips
and knees: keep the
resting foot low, at
calf or ankle height.

🖐 If you are working
on balance, bring the
resting foot to the
ankle. You can also
rest your toes on
the floor.

9   UTKATA KONASANA
Goddess or Horse Pose

This is a fun, strong, dynamic pose with lots of options.

1 From standing, step back with your right foot and turn your body to the right. Your feet should be a comfortable distance apart, so your body feels well supported. Adjust the position until it feels right for you.

2 Turn your feet out and bend into your knees, without sticking out your backside. Engage the outer edges of the feet, heels and toes and draw the inner thighs together. Your arms can be in the prayer position, out to the side, or overhead. Straighten your legs whenever you need to.

3 Alternatively, with the knees bent, shift your weight from foot to foot, moving the hips as you do so.

Benefits

🤚 Strengthens the legs and opens the inner thighs and hips.

🤚 Shifting your weight from foot to foot is great for practising balance and transitions.

Modifications

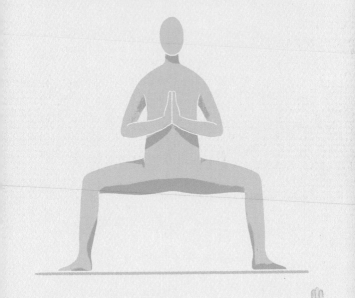

For stiff knees: avoid bending too deeply into the squat. Position the angle of the feet so that when you bend the knees, it feels comfortable.

10 SUKHASANA
Easy Sitting Pose

Despite the name, this pose is not *always* easy! See the Modifications to make it work better for you.

1 Sit on a low block or cushion, and pull the flesh back on your buttocks so that you are sitting on your sit bones.

2 Cross one shin in front of the other, with the heels moving under the opposite knee. You may find it feels more comfortable with one or the other shin in front.

3 Rest your hands on your thighs or knees, but resist pushing or pulling against the legs.

4 Sitting up tall with a long spine, find equal space in the front and back of the body. Relax your neck and shoulders.

Benefits

🖐 Strengthens the back and opens the hips and thighs.

🖐 Can bring a sense of stillness and calm, in preparation for *pranayama* or meditation.

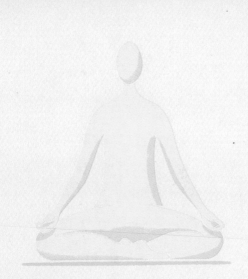

Modifications

If there is any discomfort in the hips, knees or feet, or if the knees are much higher than the hips, try the following:

 Sit on a higher block or cushion.

 Straighten out one leg slightly wider than the hip, leaving the other one folded in; keep the knee of the straight leg slightly bent.

 Straighten out both legs in front, slightly wider than the hips, with the knees slightly bent.

SUPTA MATSYENDRASANA
Reclining Twist

A wonderful restorative pose that opens the chest, upper spine and shoulders.

1 Lying on your back, roll onto your right-hand side. Bring your knees up to a right angle with your belly button. Use your right hand to hold down the thighs.

2 Open up your chest and shoulders to the ceiling and extend your left arm, palm facing up.

3 Look wherever is comfortable for your neck: straight up, to the right or to the left.

4 Breathe into any areas that feel tight: perhaps the hip, or into the upper back or chest.

5 Let the left arm, shoulder and side of the chest become heavy as they twist to the left and relax toward the floor. You can extend the right arm, too, if it feels good.

6 Repeat on the other side.

Benefits

🖐 A great counterpose for sitting at a computer.

Modifications

👋 Use a pillow to support the head, if necessary.

👋 If the twist through the torso is too much, change
the angle of the knees, or let them come away from
the floor and support them with a cushion or block.

👋 If the stretch on the extended arm/shoulder is too
strong, place a block or cushion underneath it.

SUPTA BADDHA KONASANA
Reclining Cobbler Pose

This calming and
relaxing pose opens the
front of the body. An
eye mask can feel nice
in this pose.

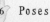

1 Lying on your back, bend your knees and bring the soles of the feet together, letting the knees fall toward the floor.

2 Lengthen the tailbone so that the lower back feels comfortable.

3 Place your hands on your belly or in line with your shoulders; alternatively, put your arms alongside your torso or take them overhead.

Benefits

🖐 Gently opens the hips and the inner thighs.

Modifications

🖐 If the stretch into the hips is too strong, place blocks or cushions under the knees.

🖐 Adjust the position of the feet, closer to or further away from the groin. Find what works for your hips and knees.

🖐 If lying flat is uncomfortable on the lower back, lie back over some cushions or bolsters, so that you are in a reclined sitting position.

SAVASANA
Corpse Pose

13

This is the most important pose, especially to end your yoga session – don't skip it! Your body temperature will drop, so you might want a blanket to cover you. An eye mask or eye bag can feel nice, especially if the room is bright.

1 Lie down on your back and make yourself comfortable: legs straight, knees bent, feet wider apart – all these are possibilities. Adjust your arms: further or closer to the torso, hands on the belly, palms up or down.

2 Allow the body to relax, sinking your weight to the floor. If you notice any areas that are holding tension, make a small adjustment or use the breath to encourage them to soften.

3 Bring your attention to your breathing, scan your body or use a guided meditation. Or simply rest! Stay like this for at least five minutes.

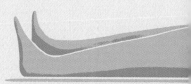

Benefits

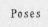 Helps the body absorb your practice: the mind–muscle connections are laid down, the nervous system is calmed, the mind stills, *prana* is stored in the body. We can rest.

Modifications

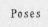 Savasana can be uncomfortable because we are unused to simple rest without distraction. If this happens, focus on your breath or use a guided meditation.

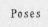 If lying down flat is uncomfortable, use pillows or try lying on your side.

Om

"Om" is a sound
and a symbol as
much as a word. It is
made up of the
sounds "AUM",
which represent the
whole of the universe
that we can pronounce
linguistically – from the A sound at
the back of the throat to the M, which finishes at the lips.

In this way "Om" represents the divine, the universe,
consciousness. For yoga in its spiritual context, "Om" is one
small way of recognizing that we are all part of something
bigger. Some teachers will chant "Om" at the start and/or
end of a class to acknowledge the universe that we explore
through yoga, as well as to celebrate the communal
consciousness and togetherness of group practice.

"Om" is said to have given rise to words such as "Hum",
"Amin" and "Amen". In this way it can simply be translated
as "Let it Be".

"*Om.*"

6.
Daily Practices

Yoga doesn't only have to be done on a mat in a classroom.
Here are some practices to use throughout your day.

1 Upon Waking

When the alarm clock goes off, it can jolt us straight into "fight or flight" mode, so that we start the day feeling stressed. This practice, from the Tantric yoga tradition, enables you to centre, ground and prepare yourself in the morning.

1 Set a timer for five to ten minutes. Find an upright seated position: in bed, with a pillow behind your back, or sitting on a cushion or chair. Make sure your spine is straight. Let your face and jaw relax, but sit with a sense of alertness: you don't want to go back to sleep.

2 Focus on your breathing. Allow it to find its natural rhythm for a few rounds, then start to lengthen it slightly, but don't force it. Breathe into your belly, lower back and chest, then exhale.

3 With your eyes closed or half open, visualize or sense a central channel through your body: from the crown of the head, following the spine, down to the pelvic floor. It goes down through your seat, the floor and into the earth; and up through the top of your head into the world. Sit for a moment with this image or feeling.

4 As you inhale, visualize or sense golden light coming up from the earth into your central channel. As you exhale,

this light goes up through the crown of the head, into the world. Repeat. If the mind wanders, you can add a mantra – such as "So" on the inhale, and "Hum" on the exhale – to help you focus.

5 When your timer goes off, release the visualization and rest. Keep the breath soft, and notice how you feel. Remain sitting with awareness for as long as necessary.

If you need a more energizing start to your day, some Sun Salutations (see page 92) or the "At Your Desk" exercises (see page 84), done standing, can be a great way to inject vitality into the body and mind before attempting the visualization.

2 At Your Desk

These practices enable you to awaken and move the body without even standing up. You can do all or a few of them, depending on the nature of your office and your work attire.

👋 Sit in an upright position, with your feet on the floor and your lower back supported. Find equal space in the front and back of the body.

👋 Move your tongue in your mouth, circle the jaw, take a big yawn, stretch and screw up your face. We hold a lot of tension in the jaw, which can translate into tension in other parts of the body. Sometimes just this "face yoga" can be enough.

👋 Start moving your shoulders: hunch them to the ears, then allow them to drop; roll them backward and forward. Allow the shoulder blades, collar bones and ribs to move with you.

👋 Rotate your elbow, wrist and finger joints; shake out your hands, flex and extend the wrists gently. This exercise is great if you do a lot of computer work.

👋 If clothing and space permit, circle through the ribcage and hips. You can also do a seated version of Cat & Cow (see page 56), softly extending and flexing the spine.

- Rotate the ankles, point the toes, flex the feet, wriggle the toes (remove your shoes, if you can).

- Place your left ankle on your right knee. If this is uncomfortable, lower the height by sliding the right foot away from you a little. Then bend slowly forward, keeping awareness in the lower back, hips and knees; if you feel any pain, sit upright. Repeat on the other side.

- Push your chair further away from your desk and fold forward, putting your hands shoulder-width apart near the edge of the desk. Gently feel as if you are lengthening your tailbone, while allowing the chest to be heavy. Stop if you feel any pain in the lower back.

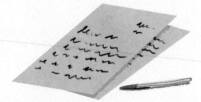

3 To De-stress

To de-stress, we need to switch our nervous system from "fight or flight" mode to "rest and restore". To do this, we need to release physical tension from the body and calm the nervous system with conscious breathing.

If you are full of nervous energy, some gentle Sun Salutations (see page 92) or the "At Your Desk" exercises (see page 84), done in a standing position, can help start the de-stressing process. Breathe deeply, and bring your mind back to your body and breath whenever you notice it wandering.

Good poses for de-stressing

Forward Fold (see page 54), Cat & Cow (see page 56), Child's Pose (see page 58), Reclining Cobbler Pose (see page 76).

When the body is still, we often become more aware of how noisy our minds are. Although we usually think we should silence our thoughts, this is very difficult to do. Instead, it can help to view our thoughts as a TV in another room – forever chattering away, but not too intrusively; all the while, focus attention on your breathing and the feelings in your body.

Deep Tummy-breathing

This practice not only gives your attention a focus, but also helps switch on your "rest and restore" mode.

1 Placing your hands on your lower belly, breathe in your natural rhythm, without force, but gently direct the breath into the space beneath your hands.

2 Pay attention to the pattern of the breath coming in and going out. Notice the way the abdomen moves up away from the spine on the inhale, and down toward the spine on the exhale. Don't force this movement; simply notice how the breath makes it happen.

As you breathe, you are massaging your vagus nerve, which travels from the gut to the brainstem, winding around your internal organs and diaphragm. This nerve switches on the relaxed, parasympathetic nervous system. Deep tummy-breathing massages this nerve, improving vagal tone – the ability to send the "rest and restore" message to the brain.

4 For Focus

Alternate nostril-breathing, or Nadi Shodhana, focuses the mind by switching the breath through alternate sides of the nose. As well as providing focus, this practice can be calming, leading to a state of relaxed alertness. Avoid it if you have a cold or a blocked nose.

1 Use your predominant hand and close the first and second fingers to the palm, leaving the thumb, ring and little fingers lifted. If you are right-handed, you will use your thumb to close the right nostril, and the ring finger to close the left.

2 Keep the eyes closed, or at least very soft and relaxed.

3 Start by closing the left nostril, and inhale through the right.

4 Close the right nostril, and exhale through the left.

5 Inhale through the left nostril.

6 Close the left nostril and exhale through the right.

7 This constitutes one round. You can repeat this for 10–20 rounds.

For added focus and concentration, you can count each inhale/exhale. For example, inhale for a count of four, exhale for a count of four.

When you have finished, pause with your eyes still closed and return to your natural breathing for a minute or so.

5 To Calm the Mind

I learned this "rooting meditation", which originates from the Indian tradition of Kashmiri Shaivism, from Alexander Filmer-Lorch. This meditation takes one to five minutes and can be done with your eyes closed or open. You can set a timer, if you wish.

1 Sit upright, with the lower back supported and feet planted, and let your tongue, jaw and eyes soften; if your eyes are open, allow the gaze to soften, too.

2 Rather than forcing the breath, find a natural rhythm and relax into the breath.

3 Bring your attention to the tip of your nose. Notice the breath in the nostrils. Watch how the breath comes in, and visualize it going to the top of your head. As you breathe out, see the breath travel down the spine into the lower back. Return to the tip of your nose: inhaling, the breath goes to the top of the head; exhaling, it goes down the spine. Repeat.

4 Keep the breath and the eyes soft. Visualize the breath travelling up and down. Don't rush your breath. Notice any tendencies to force or push it; allow the flow of breath to be easy, as far as possible.

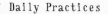

5 As you exhale, let the sensation of your breath collect in the lower body, offering a grounding sensation.

6 Repeat as many times as feels comfortable. Then stop the visualization and just sit, with your attention resting behind your eyes, and soft breathing. Come out of the meditation when you are ready.

If you feel anxious during the meditation, stop and perhaps do some of the "At Your Desk" exercises (see page 84) to help calm the nervous system.

6 To Energize

You can take this Sun Salutation variation slowly and pause in each pose, or move with your breath. Repeat as many times as you like, leading equal times with each leg.

1 From Tadasana (see page 52), bend the knees and roll down into Forward Fold (see page 54).

2 With your hands on the floor, step the right leg back and bring the knee to the floor. Lift into a Low Lunge (see page 62).

3 Bring the hands to the floor and step back into Down Dog (see page 60) to prepare for step 4a **OR** 4b.

4a <u>Waving Vinyasa</u> (on hands and feet)

- Bend the knees, bringing your hips toward your heels.
- Push through the toes, rounding your back and looking at your belly, in a long Cat Pose (see page 57).
- As your shoulders arrive over your wrists, lower the pelvis toward the floor, but keep the chest lifted. You are now in Upward-facing Dog.
- Push through the hands and feet to come up, rounding the back and looking at your belly. As you move back, soften the knees as you arrive in Down Dog.

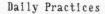

4b <u>Baby Wave</u> (on hands and knees)

- Start on all fours. Tuck your toes and move your hips back toward your heels. Take the arms further out in front, so they are straight and active.
- Push through your toes to come up into Cat Pose.
- As your shoulders arrive over the wrists, bring the hips forward as far as feels comfortable. The arms stay straight, the chest lifted. The knees can come up from the floor.
- Push through the hands and feet, rounding your back and looking at your belly.
- As you move back, soften the knees, push through your heels and come up into Down Dog.

5 Step the right foot forward between the hands (or bring both knees to the floor and step the right foot forward).

6 Bring the back knee down and lift the chest into a Low Lunge (see page 62).

7 As the hands come to the floor, tuck the back toes, lift the back knee and push off the toes to step the back foot forward: you are now in Forward Fold.

8 Roll up to standing. Repeat with the left leg leading.

7 Before Bed

All these poses can be done on your bed.

Seated Forward Fold

1 Sitting on your pillows, with the legs slightly wider than the hips, place another pillow or cushion under the knees.

2 Bend forward and drape yourself over your bent knees. You can support the head with more pillows or with your hands.

3 Breathe into the back of the body.

Lying-down Tree

1 Lying flat, keep the left leg straight and bring the sole of the right foot against the inside of the straight leg. You can use a pillow to support the right knee.

2 Repeat on the other side.

Reclining Twist (see page 74)

Legs-up-the-Wall Pose

1 Sit sideways on your pillows, then swing your legs round, up against the headboard or wall, with your torso lying on the bed.

Deep Tummy-breathing (see page 87)

This can be done lying down or with your legs up the wall.

Acknowledgments

With thanks to

Alexander Filmer-Lorch, author of *Inside Meditation* and *The Inner Power of Stillness,* for the meditation on page 91

Angus Ford Robertson of Battersea Yoga

Sally Kempton, author of *Awakening Shakti,* for her teachings on meditation

James Mallinson and Mark Singleton, authors of *Roots of Yoga,* for their teachings on the history of yoga

Julie Martin of Brahmani Yoga

Lucy Parker of Flow Tunbridge Wells

Christopher Hareesh Wallis, author of *Tantra Illuminated* and *The Recognition Sutras*, for the meditation on page 82

Bridget Woods Kramer of BWK Yoga

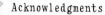